CONTENTS

CHAPTER 1: INTRODUCTION

As individuals age, maintaining a safe and secure living environment becomes paramount to ensure their well-being and quality of life. This chapter sets the stage for the book by highlighting the critical importance of home safety for seniors, providing insightful statistics on common accidents and injuries among this demographic, and outlining the primary goal of the book — promoting a safer living environment for seniors.

1.1 Importance of Home Safety for Seniors

Home is a sanctuary, a place where one should feel secure and comfortable. For seniors, whose mobility and health may be more vulnerable, the significance of a safe home environment cannot be overstated. The home serves as the primary setting for daily activities, and a safe living space directly impacts the physical, mental, and emotional well-being of seniors.

This section delves into the various aspects of a home that contribute to safety, from well-lit pathways to secure flooring, and how these elements collectively foster independence and confidence among seniors. It emphasizes that creating a safe home is not only about accident prevention but also about preserving a sense of autonomy and dignity for the elderly.

1.2 Statistics on Common Accidents and Injuries Among Seniors

To underscore the need for a focus on home safety, this section presents compelling statistics on the prevalence of accidents and injuries among seniors. Common incidents, such as falls, burns, and medication-related issues, are explored with an emphasis on how these events can lead to serious consequences for the elderly population.

By providing concrete data, the chapter aims to raise awareness about the vulnerability of seniors to accidents within their homes. This statistical insight serves as a compelling motivation for readers to take proactive steps in making their homes safer, thereby reducing the risks associated with aging in place.

1.3 The Goal of the Book: Promoting a Safer Living Environment

This section outlines the overarching objective of the book — to empower seniors and their caregivers with the knowledge and resources needed to create a secure living environment. It highlights the proactive approach the book takes in addressing potential safety concerns, offering practical advice, and guiding readers through the process of enhancing home safety.

The goal is not just to impart information but to inspire action. By the end of the book, readers should feel confident in implementing changes within their homes to mitigate potential risks. Whether through home modifications, awareness of common hazards, or adopting safety protocols, the book aims to be a comprehensive guide for seniors and their support networks in fostering a living space that prioritizes safety without compromising independence.

CHAPTER 2: ASSESSING HOME HAZARDS

As seniors age, the home that once felt familiar and secure may gradually become a source of potential hazards. Conducting a comprehensive home safety assessment is a proactive and essential step in ensuring that the living environment remains conducive to the well-being and independence of seniors. This chapter delves into the intricacies of home hazard assessments, guiding readers through the process of identifying potential dangers in different areas of the home and emphasizing the importance of regular assessments as mobility and health conditions evolve.

2.1 The Need for a Comprehensive Home Safety Assessment

A home safety assessment is not merely a checklist of tasks; it is a holistic examination of the living space to identify and address potential hazards that could compromise the safety of seniors. This section emphasizes the need for a thorough and comprehensive assessment, one that goes beyond the obvious dangers to consider the unique needs and challenges faced by each individual.

Readers are encouraged to approach the assessment with a proactive mindset, viewing it as a tool for enhancing the overall quality of life for seniors. The assessment encompasses various dimensions, including physical safety, accessibility, and emotional well-being, making it a valuable resource for tailoring safety measures to the specific requirements of the elderly residents.

2.2 Identifying Potential Hazards in Different Areas of the Home

This section provides a detailed exploration of potential hazards in different areas of the home, offering practical insights into common safety concerns and how to address them. The goal is to empower readers with the knowledge to recognize and mitigate risks, creating a safer living environment for seniors.

- **Living Room and Common Areas:**
  - Evaluation of furniture placement for ease of navigation.
  - Identification of tripping hazards, such as loose rugs or clutter.
  - Ensuring adequate lighting to prevent falls and enhance visibility.

- **Kitchen:**
  - Assessment of countertop heights and ease of access to appliances.
  - Strategies for organizing kitchen items to minimize the risk of accidents.
  - Fire safety measures, including the proper use and placement of kitchen appliances.

- **Bedroom:**
  - Considerations for a comfortable and accessible bed.
  - Adequate lighting for nighttime navigation.
  - Prevention of bedroom-specific hazards like tangled cords or obstructed pathways.

- **Bathroom:**
  - Installation of grab bars and non-slip surfaces in the shower and near the toilet.
  - Evaluation of the accessibility of bathroom fixtures.
  - Strategies for maintaining a dry and safe bathroom environment.

- **Stairways and Hallways:**
  - Assessment of handrails and banisters for stability.
  - Strategies for reducing tripping hazards on stairs.
  - Adequate lighting in stairwells and hallways.
- **Outdoor Areas:**
  - Evaluation of pathways and entrances for accessibility.
  - Considerations for outdoor lighting and visibility.
  - Strategies for creating a secure outdoor environment.

By breaking down potential hazards in this manner, readers gain a practical understanding of how to conduct a systematic assessment of their homes, fostering a proactive approach to safety.

2.3 Importance of Regular Assessments as Mobility and Health Change

One of the key messages in this section is the dynamic nature of home safety needs for seniors. Mobility and health conditions can evolve over time, necessitating regular reassessments of the living environment. The chapter underscores that what may be a safe arrangement today might not remain so in the future.

Readers are encouraged to incorporate regular home safety assessments into their routine, adapting their living spaces to changing circumstances. This not only involves physical changes, such as installing additional grab bars or ramps, but also considering modifications based on evolving health conditions. For instance, as mobility decreases, adjustments may be needed to ensure a seamless and safe living experience.

The chapter emphasizes that home safety is an ongoing

process, not a one-time task. By regularly reassessing the home environment, seniors and their caregivers can stay ahead of potential hazards, fostering a living space that adapts to the changing needs of its occupants.

In conclusion, Chapter 2 serves as a comprehensive guide to home safety assessments for seniors. It instills the importance of a thorough evaluation, provides practical insights into identifying hazards in different areas of the home, and stresses the dynamic nature of home safety, urging readers to make regular assessments a crucial part of their caregiving routine.

CHAPTER 3: FALL PREVENTION

Falls among seniors can have profound consequences, affecting not only physical health but also mental well-being and overall quality of life. This chapter delves into the nuances of fall prevention, offering a comprehensive understanding of the impact of falls on seniors, practical tips for preventing falls through home modifications, and exercises designed to improve balance and reduce the risk of falls.

3.1 Understanding the Impact of Falls on Seniors

Falls represent a significant health risk for seniors, with far-reaching consequences that extend beyond the immediate physical injuries. This section explores the multifaceted impact of falls on seniors, addressing both the physical and psychological aspects.

- **Physical Consequences:**
    - Fractures, particularly hip fractures, which can severely impact mobility.
    - Sprains, strains, and other musculoskeletal injuries.
    - Head injuries, including concussions, which may have long-term cognitive effects.

- **Psychological Consequences:**
    - Fear of falling, leading to reduced physical activity and social isolation.
    - Anxiety and depression resulting from the loss of confidence in one's ability to move safely.
    - Decreased overall quality of life due to the limitations imposed by the fear of falling.

Understanding the full spectrum of consequences is crucial for seniors and their caregivers. It not only highlights the importance of proactive fall prevention but also motivates individuals to take concrete steps to mitigate the risks associated with falls.

3.2 Tips for Preventing Falls Through Home Modifications

This section provides practical tips and guidelines for modifying the home environment to minimize fall risks. The goal is to create a living space that supports mobility and independence while significantly reducing the likelihood of accidents.

- **Flooring and Carpets:**
    - Securing carpets and rugs to prevent tripping.
    - Opting for non-slip flooring in areas prone to moisture, such as the bathroom and kitchen.

- **Lighting:**
    - Ensuring adequate lighting throughout the home, especially in hallways and staircases.
    - Installing motion-activated lights to enhance visibility during nighttime movements.

- **Furniture Arrangement:**
    - Rearranging furniture to create clear and unobstructed pathways.
    - Removing clutter and unnecessary items to reduce the risk of tripping.

- **Bathroom Safety:**
    - Installing grab bars near the toilet and in the shower.
    - Using non-slip mats and adhesive strips to prevent slips in the bathroom.

- **Stair Safety:**
    - Securing handrails on both sides of staircases.
    - Applying contrasting colors to the edge of stairs

for better visibility.

- **Footwear:**
  - Encouraging the use of supportive and non-slip footwear.
  - Discouraging the use of high heels or shoes with inadequate traction.

By implementing these modifications, seniors can significantly reduce the environmental factors that contribute to falls within the home.

3.3 Exercises to Improve Balance and Reduce the Risk of Falls

Physical activity plays a crucial role in fall prevention by enhancing strength, balance, and flexibility. This section introduces a series of exercises tailored to improve these key elements, thereby reducing the risk of falls.

- **Strength Exercises:**
  - Leg lifts to strengthen the muscles in the thighs.
  - Arm raises to enhance upper body strength.
  - Core exercises to improve overall stability.

- **Balance Exercises:**
  - Heel-to-toe walking to promote balance and coordination.
  - Standing on one leg with support for gradual balance improvement.
  - Tai Chi, a low-impact exercise known for enhancing balance and flexibility.

- **Flexibility Exercises:**
  - Neck and shoulder stretches to maintain flexibility in the upper body.
  - Ankle circles and toe taps to promote flexibility in the lower extremities.

- Yoga poses focusing on gentle stretching and balance.

The chapter stresses the importance of consulting with healthcare professionals before starting any exercise routine, ensuring that the chosen activities align with individual health conditions and fitness levels.

In conclusion, Chapter 3 serves as a comprehensive guide to fall prevention for seniors. It delves into the far-reaching consequences of falls, provides practical tips for home modifications to minimize risks, and introduces a range of exercises designed to improve balance and overall physical well-being. By combining environmental modifications with targeted exercises, seniors can actively reduce the risk of falls and maintain a safer and more independent lifestyle.

CHAPTER 4: HOME MODIFICATIONS

Creating an age-friendly living space is pivotal to ensuring the safety and independence of seniors at home. This chapter delves into the intricate details of home modifications, providing comprehensive guidance on adapting the living environment to meet the unique needs of the elderly. From installing grab bars to incorporating technological solutions, the chapter explores practical strategies to make homes safer for seniors.

4.1 The Rationale Behind Home Modifications

Before delving into specific modifications, it's essential to establish the rationale behind adapting the home environment for seniors. Aging often brings changes in mobility, vision, and overall physical health, necessitating adjustments to the living space. This section explores the reasons for home modifications, emphasizing the proactive nature of these changes to enhance the quality of life for seniors.

- **Preserving Independence:**
    - Adapting the home allows seniors to maintain autonomy and independence in their daily activities.
    - Modifications reduce the reliance on caregivers, fostering a sense of self-sufficiency.

- **Preventing Accidents:**
    - Home modifications address potential hazards, minimizing the risk of accidents such as falls.
    - A safer environment contributes to the overall well-being and peace of mind for both seniors and their caregivers.

- **Supporting Aging in Place:**
    - By making the home more age-friendly, seniors can continue living in a familiar and comfortable environment.
    - Modifications contribute to the feasibility of aging in place, avoiding the need for institutional care.

4.2 Key Home Modifications for Senior Safety

This section provides an in-depth exploration of specific home modifications, offering practical insights into how each adaptation contributes to creating a safer living space for seniors.

- **Grab Bars and Handrails:**
    - Proper placement of grab bars in bathrooms and areas prone to slipping.
    - Installation of handrails along staircases and hallways to provide support.

- **Ramps and Elevators:**
    - Building ramps for wheelchair accessibility, especially at entrances.
    - Considering the installation of residential elevators for multi-story homes.

- **Accessible Flooring:**
    - Choosing flooring materials that reduce the risk of slips and falls.
    - Eliminating tripping hazards by securing carpets and rugs.

- **Bathroom Modifications:**
    - Installing walk-in showers with non-slip flooring.
    - Utilizing raised toilet seats and grab bars for enhanced bathroom safety.

- **Kitchen Adaptations:**
    - Lowering countertop heights to accommodate wheelchair users.
    - Opting for easy-to-reach storage solutions for kitchen utensils and supplies.

- **Lighting Solutions:**
    - Ensuring ample lighting throughout the home, especially in high-traffic areas.
    - Utilizing motion-activated lights to enhance visibility during nighttime movements.

- **Smart Home Technologies:**
    - Incorporating technologies such as smart doorbells and security cameras for enhanced safety.
    - Using voice-activated devices to control lighting, temperature, and security features.

- **Comfortable Furniture:**
    - Choosing ergonomic furniture that supports proper posture and ease of use.
    - Ensuring that chairs and sofas have appropriate height and support for seniors.

4.3 Financial Considerations and Resources

While the importance of home modifications is clear, this section addresses the financial aspect of implementing these changes. It explores potential funding sources, government assistance programs, and available resources to help seniors and their caregivers navigate the financial considerations associated with home modifications.

- **Government Assistance Programs:**
    - Overview of programs that provide financial aid for home modifications.

- Guidance on eligibility criteria and application processes.
- **Community Resources:**
    - Local organizations and charities that offer assistance with home modifications.
    - Utilizing community resources to access affordable or free services.
- **Insurance Coverage:**
    - Exploring insurance options that may cover certain home modifications.
    - Understanding the limitations and requirements of insurance coverage.

This section empowers readers with information on how to make home modifications within budgetary constraints, ensuring that creating a safe living environment is feasible for a wide range of individuals.

4.4 Home Modification Planning and Implementation

Creating a plan for home modifications is a crucial step in ensuring a seamless and effective process. This section provides a step-by-step guide on planning and implementing home modifications, from assessing individual needs to finding qualified professionals for the job.

- **Assessment of Individual Needs:**
    - Understanding the specific requirements of the senior resident.
    - Identifying priority areas for modification based on individual mobility and health considerations.
- **Consultation with Professionals:**
    - Engaging with occupational therapists and home modification specialists.

- Seeking professional advice on the most effective and personalized modifications.

- **Budgeting and Cost Estimates:**
    - Creating a realistic budget for home modifications.
    - Obtaining cost estimates from contractors and service providers.

- **Project Timeline:**
    - Developing a timeline for the phased implementation of modifications.
    - Considering temporary housing arrangements during significant renovations.

By providing a comprehensive guide to planning and implementing home modifications, this section empowers readers to take practical steps toward creating a safer living space for seniors.

In conclusion, Chapter 4 serves as a detailed roadmap for home modifications tailored to the needs of seniors. It underscores the rationale behind these adaptations, explores key modifications, addresses financial considerations, and provides a practical guide for planning and implementation. By making the home environment more age-friendly, seniors can enjoy a heightened sense of security, independence, and overall well-being.

CHAPTER 5: MEDICATION MANAGEMENT

As seniors age, managing medications becomes increasingly crucial for maintaining health and well-being. This chapter delves into the intricacies of medication management for seniors, emphasizing the importance of a systematic approach to medication adherence and safety. From organizing medications to understanding potential risks and interactions, this chapter provides comprehensive guidance for both seniors and their caregivers.

5.1 The Importance of Medication Management for Seniors

Managing medications effectively is a critical aspect of senior healthcare. This section explores the significance of medication management, highlighting how it contributes to overall health, prevents complications, and ensures that seniors receive the intended benefits from their prescribed medications.

- **Adherence and Treatment Efficacy:**
    - The impact of consistent medication adherence on the effectiveness of treatment.
    - The role of medication management in preventing missed doses and potential complications.

- **Preventing Adverse Reactions:**
    - The potential risks of medication interactions and adverse reactions.
    - How proper medication management minimizes the likelihood of adverse effects.

- **Maintaining Independence:**

- The link between effective medication management and the ability to live independently.
- Empowering seniors to take an active role in managing their medications.

5.2 Tips for Organizing and Managing Medications

This section provides practical tips and strategies for organizing medications to ensure accuracy, timeliness, and adherence. It addresses common challenges seniors face in managing multiple medications and offers solutions to streamline the process.

- **Medication Scheduling:**
  - Creating a consistent daily routine for taking medications.
  - Utilizing pill organizers or smartphone apps to set reminders.

- **Labeling and Identification:**
  - Ensuring clear labeling of medications, including dosage instructions.
  - Using color-coded pill organizers or blister packs for easy identification.

- **Storage Guidelines:**
  - Proper storage of medications to maintain potency and safety.
  - Guidelines for storing medications that require refrigeration.

- **Medication Reviews:**
  - The importance of regular medication reviews with healthcare providers.
  - Discussing potential side effects, interactions, and adjustments to the medication regimen.

5.3 Understanding Potential Risks of Medication Interactions

Seniors often manage multiple medications simultaneously, increasing the risk of interactions and adverse effects. This section provides an in-depth exploration of potential risks associated with medication interactions and offers guidance on how to minimize these risks.

- **Polypharmacy Awareness:**
  - Defining polypharmacy and its implications for seniors.
  - Strategies for reducing unnecessary medications and simplifying the medication regimen.

- **Communication with Healthcare Providers:**
  - Encouraging open communication with healthcare providers about all medications.
  - Providing a comprehensive list of prescribed medications, over-the-counter drugs, and supplements.

- **Monitoring for Side Effects:**
  - Understanding common side effects of medications.
  - Knowing when to seek medical attention for unexpected reactions.

5.4 Educating Seniors on Safe Medication Practices

This section focuses on empowering seniors with knowledge about safe medication practices. It emphasizes the importance of proactive communication with healthcare providers, understanding medication instructions, and being vigilant about potential risks.

- **Reading Medication Labels:**
  - Guidance on interpreting medication labels, including dosage, frequency, and special

instructions.

- Encouraging the use of magnifiers or reading glasses if needed.

- **Questioning Medication Changes:**
    - Advocating for seniors to ask questions about new medications or changes to existing ones.
    - Seeking clarification on potential side effects and interactions.

- **Utilizing Medication Management Tools:**
    - Introducing seniors to tools such as pill organizers, medication reminder apps, and automated dispensing systems.
    - Providing step-by-step tutorials on using these tools effectively.

5.5 The Role of Caregivers in Medication Management

Caregivers play a crucial role in supporting seniors with medication management. This section addresses the responsibilities of caregivers, offering guidance on effective communication, coordination with healthcare providers, and monitoring for potential issues.

- **Open Communication:**
    - The importance of transparent communication between seniors, caregivers, and healthcare providers.
    - Encouraging an open dialogue about any difficulties or concerns related to medications.

- **Coordination with Healthcare Providers:**
    - The role of caregivers in facilitating communication with healthcare professionals.
    - Collaborating with healthcare providers to ensure a unified approach to medication

management.

- **Regular Medication Reviews:**
    - Establishing a routine for regular medication reviews with healthcare providers.
    - Advocating for seniors during medical appointments to address any medication-related concerns.

5.6 Seeking Professional Guidance for Medication Management

For complex medication regimens or instances where seniors face challenges in self-managing medications, seeking professional guidance becomes crucial. This section explores the role of pharmacists, geriatric care managers, and other healthcare professionals in providing specialized assistance.

- **Pharmacist Consultations:**
    - The benefits of scheduling regular consultations with pharmacists.
    - Leveraging the expertise of pharmacists for medication reconciliation and guidance.

- **Geriatric Care Managers:**
    - Exploring the role of geriatric care managers in coordinating healthcare services, including medication management.
    - Utilizing the services of geriatric care managers for comprehensive care planning.

- **Home Healthcare Services:**
    - Considering home healthcare services for seniors who require hands-on assistance with medication administration.
    - Discussing the potential benefits of medication management support from trained professionals.

5.7 Incorporating Technological Solutions for Medication Management

This section introduces the role of technology in enhancing medication management for seniors. It explores the use of smartphone apps, electronic pill dispensers, and other digital tools that can simplify the process and improve adherence.

- **Medication Reminder Apps:**
    - Overview of smartphone apps designed to send reminders for medication doses.
    - Tips for selecting and using medication reminder apps effectively.

- **Automated Dispensing Systems:**
    - Exploring electronic pill dispensers that organize and dispense medications according to a preset schedule.
    - Guidelines for selecting automated dispensing systems based on individual needs.

- **Telehealth Services:**
    - The potential of telehealth services in medication management, including virtual consultations with healthcare providers.
    - Considerations for seniors who may benefit from remote medication monitoring.

5.8 Adapting Medication Management to Evolving Health Conditions

As health conditions evolve, so do medication needs. This section emphasizes the importance of regularly reassessing medication management strategies to align with changes in health status, ensuring that the medication regimen remains safe and effective.

- **Health Condition Changes:**
    - Recognizing the impact of evolving health conditions on medication requirements.
    - The importance of promptly informing healthcare providers about changes in health status.

- **Adjusting Medication Schedules:**
    - Strategies for adapting medication schedules to accommodate changes in daily routines or sleeping patterns.
    - Coordination with healthcare providers to modify dosages or frequencies as needed.

5.9 Integrating Medication Management into Overall Health and Wellness

This section emphasizes the interconnectedness of medication management with overall health and wellness. It explores lifestyle factors, nutrition, and exercise as integral components that can complement effective medication management for seniors.

- **Nutrition and Medication Interactions:**
    - The impact of dietary choices on medication absorption and effectiveness.
    - Consulting with healthcare providers about potential interactions between medications and specific foods.

- **Exercise and Medication Effects:**
    - The role of physical activity in supporting overall health and potentially influencing medication effectiveness.
    - Customizing exercise routines

CHAPTER 6: FIRE AND ELECTRICAL SAFETY

Ensuring the safety of seniors at home involves a comprehensive approach that extends beyond physical well-being to include protection from potential hazards such as fires and electrical accidents. This chapter delves into the critical aspects of fire and electrical safety, addressing guidelines for fire prevention, emergency evacuation plans, electrical safety tips, and the importance of proactive measures to safeguard seniors in their living environments.

6.1 Importance of Fire Prevention and Emergency Preparedness

This section lays the foundation for understanding the significance of fire prevention and emergency preparedness for seniors. Fires can pose a significant threat to the safety of individuals, and seniors, in particular, may face additional challenges in responding to emergencies. The discussion explores how proactive measures can mitigate these risks and create a safer living environment.

- **Vulnerabilities of Seniors:**

    - Recognizing factors that may make seniors more vulnerable during fires, such as reduced mobility or impaired hearing.

    - Highlighting the importance of tailored fire prevention strategies for this demographic.

- **Impact on Overall Safety:**
    - Discussing the ripple effect of fire incidents on the overall safety and well-being of seniors.
        - Emphasizing the role of prevention in

maintaining a secure living space.

- **Empowering Seniors:**
  - Encouraging seniors to actively participate in fire prevention and emergency preparedness efforts.
  - Providing resources and information to empower them to take charge of their safety.

6.2 Guidelines for Fire Prevention

Fire prevention is a critical component of home safety for seniors. This section provides comprehensive guidelines on minimizing fire risks within the home environment, from identifying potential hazards to adopting preventive measures.

- **Safe Cooking Practices:**
  - Emphasizing the importance of attentive cooking habits.
  - Tips for using kitchen appliances safely and avoiding distractions while cooking.

- **Electrical Appliance Safety:**
  - Guidelines for the proper use and maintenance of electrical appliances.
  - Identifying signs of wear and tear in cords and plugs, and promptly addressing issues.

- **Heating Safety:**
  - Safe use of space heaters and other heating devices.
  - Ensuring proper ventilation and clearance around heating sources.

- **Smoking Safety:**
  - Encouraging smoking outdoors and providing safe disposal methods for smoking materials.
  - Implementing strict no-smoking policies in

bedrooms and other enclosed spaces.

- **Candle Safety:**
    - Alternatives to traditional candles for ambient lighting.
    - Safe practices when using candles, including keeping them away from flammable materials.

- **Fireplace Safety:**
    - Ensuring proper maintenance and inspection of fireplaces.
    - Guidelines for safe use, including using screens and monitoring sparks.

6.3 Emergency Evacuation Planning

Preparing for emergencies, including the need for evacuation, is crucial for seniors. This section guides readers through the process of developing effective emergency evacuation plans tailored to the unique needs of older individuals.

- **Accessible Escape Routes:**
    - Identifying accessible escape routes from different areas of the home.
    - Ensuring clear pathways to exits and avoiding clutter.

- **Emergency Exit Assistance:**
    - Establishing communication plans for seeking assistance during evacuations.
    - Collaborating with neighbors, friends, or local services for support.

- **Evacuation Kits:**
    - Creating personalized evacuation kits with essential items such as medications, important documents, and emergency contact information.

- Regularly updating kits to reflect changing needs and circumstances.

- **Communication Protocols:**
  - Establishing clear communication protocols within the household during emergencies.
  - Utilizing communication devices and systems that cater to seniors' preferences and abilities.

Electrical Safety Tips for Seniors

Electrical safety is integral to preventing accidents and fires in the home. This section provides practical tips for seniors to enhance electrical safety, covering areas such as appliance use, electrical system maintenance, and precautions against electrical shocks.

- **Appliance Maintenance:**
  - Regular inspection and maintenance of electrical appliances.
  - Prompt replacement or repair of malfunctioning appliances.

- **Proper Use of Extension Cords:**
  - Guidelines for the safe use of extension cords, including avoiding overloading outlets.
  - Using extension cords with surge protection features.

- **Electrical System Inspection:**
  - Periodic inspection of the electrical system by qualified professionals.
  - Addressing any signs of wear, damage, or outdated components.

- **Safety with Outlets and Plugs:**
  - Ensuring the proper fit of plugs in outlets to prevent sparks.
  - Use of outlet covers to protect against

accidental contact.

- **Use of Space Heaters:**
    - Safe practices when using space heaters, including maintaining distance from combustible materials.
    - Turning off space heaters when not in use or when sleeping.

6.5 Importance of Smoke Detectors and Fire Extinguishers

Smoke detectors and fire extinguishers are critical tools for early fire detection and intervention. This section highlights their importance, providing guidance on proper installation, maintenance, and usage.

- **Smoke Detector Placement:**
    - Strategic placement of smoke detectors in key areas of the home, including bedrooms and hallways.
    - Regular testing and battery replacement to ensure functionality.
- **Understanding Smoke Detector Alerts:**
    - Educating seniors on the different alert sounds and what each signifies.
    - Immediate response protocols when a smoke detector is triggered.
- **Types of Fire Extinguishers:**
    - Overview of different types of fire extinguishers and their uses.
    - Guidelines on selecting the appropriate fire extinguisher for different types of fires.
- **Proper Fire Extinguisher Usage:**
    - Training seniors on the proper technique for using fire extinguishers.

- Encouraging periodic practice sessions for familiarization.

6.6 Addressing Specific Challenges for Seniors in Fire and Electrical Safety

Seniors may face specific challenges that require tailored solutions in fire and electrical safety. This section addresses these challenges and provides practical strategies for mitigating risks.

- **Hearing Impairment:**
    - Utilizing visual and tactile alerts in addition to auditory alarms.
    - Incorporating bed shakers or vibrating devices for notification.

- **Limited Mobility:**
    - Customizing evacuation plans to accommodate limited mobility.
    - Identifying alternative safe areas within the home in case of evacuation difficulties.

- **Cognitive Impairments:**
    - Implementing simple and easily recognizable signage for emergency routes.
    - Engaging in regular drills and practice sessions to enhance familiarity.

Regular Maintenance and Inspections

Ensuring the ongoing effectiveness of fire and electrical safety measures requires regular maintenance and inspections. This section provides guidance on establishing routines for checking equipment, conducting inspections, and addressing issues promptly.

- **Scheduled Checklists:**
    - Creating checklists for routine inspections of smoke detectors, electrical systems, and fire

extinguishers.

- Incorporating these checklists into overall home safety routines.

- **Professional Inspections:**
    - Arranging for professional inspections of electrical systems and appliances.
    - Scheduling regular assessments of the home's fire safety features.

- **Documentation and Records:**
    - Maintaining records of inspections, repairs, and equipment replacements.
    - Storing important safety-related documentation in accessible locations.

6.8 Educational Initiatives for Seniors and Caregivers

- Educational initiatives play a crucial role in promoting fire and electrical safety among seniors and their caregivers. This section explores various methods of dissemination, including workshops, informational materials, and

-

CHAPTER 7: CREATING A SUPPORTIVE SOCIAL ENVIRONMENT

As seniors age, maintaining a vibrant social life becomes integral to their overall well-being. This chapter explores the importance of fostering a supportive social environment for seniors, addressing the benefits of social connections, strategies for overcoming social isolation, and creating inclusive communities that enhance the quality of life for older individuals.

7.1 The Impact of Social Connections on Senior Well-being

This section delves into the multifaceted impact of social connections on the well-being of seniors. It highlights the physical, emotional, and cognitive benefits that stem from maintaining an active and supportive social life.

- **Physical Health:**
    - Studies on the positive correlation between social engagement and physical health.
    - The role of social interactions in reducing the risk of chronic illnesses and promoting longevity.

- **Emotional Well-being:**
    - The impact of social connections on emotional resilience and mental health.
    - How supportive social networks contribute to a sense of purpose and fulfillment.

- **Cognitive Benefits:**
    - Research on the cognitive benefits of social engagement, including lower rates of cognitive

decline.

- The role of stimulating conversations and activities in maintaining cognitive function.

7.2 Recognizing and Addressing Social Isolation

Social isolation can have detrimental effects on seniors, impacting both their physical and mental health. This section explores the signs of social isolation, its contributing factors, and strategies for recognizing and addressing this prevalent issue.

- **Signs of Social Isolation:**
  - Identifying indicators such as withdrawal from social activities, increased loneliness, and a decline in overall mood.
  - Recognizing the impact of life changes, health conditions, or mobility issues on social connections.

- **Contributing Factors:**
  - Understanding common factors contributing to social isolation, including loss of loved ones, retirement, or relocation.
  - Recognizing the role of societal attitudes and ageism in perpetuating isolation.

- **Strategies for Overcoming Isolation:**
  - Encouraging seniors to explore new social opportunities, such as clubs, classes, or volunteer activities.
  - Facilitating connections through technology, including virtual meet-ups with friends and family.

7.3 Building Inclusive Communities for Seniors

Creating communities that embrace and support seniors is crucial for their social well-being. This section explores the concept of age-friendly communities, focusing on urban planning, social programs, and initiatives that foster inclusivity.

- **Accessible Public Spaces:**
    - Urban planning strategies to create accessible parks, recreational areas, and walking paths for seniors.
    - The importance of designing public spaces that accommodate diverse mobility levels.

- **Senior-Friendly Events and Programs:**
    - Initiatives that cater to the interests and needs of seniors, including cultural events, workshops, and fitness programs.
    - Creating age-inclusive spaces that promote intergenerational interactions.

- **Transportation Accessibility:**
    - Ensuring that public transportation is accessible and accommodating for seniors.
    - Implementing senior-friendly transportation options, such as shuttle services or community transport programs.

7.4 Technology as a Social Connector

Technology plays a pivotal role in connecting seniors with the broader community and fostering social interactions. This section explores the benefits of technology, addressing potential barriers and providing guidance on incorporating digital tools into the social lives of seniors.

- **Social Media and Communication Platforms:**
    - The role of social media in facilitating connections with friends, family, and community groups.
    - Exploring user-friendly communication platforms for video calls, messaging, and

virtual gatherings.

- **Online Learning and Hobbies:**
    - Access to online courses, workshops, and hobby groups that cater to seniors' interests.
    - Utilizing technology to explore new hobbies, such as virtual book clubs, art classes, or gardening forums.

- **Telehealth and Remote Services:**
    - The convenience of telehealth services for medical consultations and healthcare monitoring.
    - Utilizing technology to access remote services, including grocery delivery, fitness classes, and virtual support groups.

7.5 Family and Intergenerational Bonds

The chapter delves into the importance of family and intergenerational bonds in creating a supportive social environment for seniors. It explores the reciprocal benefits of these connections and offers insights into maintaining strong familial ties.

- **Quality Time with Family:**
    - Strategies for fostering meaningful interactions with family members.
    - The importance of open communication and shared activities.

- **Involvement in Grandparenting:**
    - Exploring the unique role of seniors in the lives of their grandchildren.
    - Encouraging activities that strengthen the bond between grandparents and grandchildren.

- **Intergenerational Programs:**
  - Participating in community programs that promote interactions between different age groups.
  - The mutual benefits of intergenerational relationships in fostering understanding and empathy.

7.6 Volunteering and Civic Engagement

Engaging in volunteer activities and civic participation not only provides seniors with a sense of purpose but also connects them with the broader community. This section explores the positive impact of volunteering and provides guidance on finding meaningful opportunities.

- **Benefits of Volunteering:**
  - Enhancing self-esteem and sense of accomplishment through contributing to others.
  - The positive effects of volunteering on mental health and overall life satisfaction.

- **Finding Suitable Volunteer Opportunities:**
  - Exploring volunteer opportunities aligned with seniors' skills, interests, and time availability.
  - The role of local organizations and volunteer coordinators in connecting seniors with suitable programs.

- **Civic Engagement Initiatives:**
  - Encouraging seniors to participate in local civic activities, community meetings, and advocacy.
  - The empowerment that comes from actively contributing to community decisions and initiatives.

7.7 Supportive Caregiving Networks

Caregiving networks play a pivotal role in the social well-being of seniors, providing essential support and companionship. This section explores the dynamics of caregiving relationships, addressing both formal and informal caregiving structures.

- **Formal Caregiving Services:**
    - Utilizing professional caregiving services, including in-home care, respite care, and companionship services.
    - The importance of clear communication and collaboration between seniors, family members, and caregivers.

- **Informal Caregiving Networks:**
    - The role of family members, friends, and neighbors in informal caregiving networks.
    - Strategies for building and maintaining strong support systems.

- **Respite Care for Caregivers:**
    - Recognizing the challenges faced by caregivers and the importance of respite care.
    - Creating plans for temporary relief to prevent caregiver burnout.

7.8 Cultural and Recreational Opportunities

Cultural and recreational activities contribute significantly to the social enrichment of seniors. This section explores the diverse opportunities available, from cultural events to recreational pursuits, and encourages seniors to explore activities aligned with their interests.

- **Cultural Outings and Events:**
    - Participating in cultural outings, museum visits, and art exhibitions.

- The role of cultural events in fostering a sense of connection and shared experiences.

- **Recreational Clubs and Hobbies:**
    - Joining recreational clubs, hobby groups, or sports leagues.
    - The benefits of shared interests in forming social bonds.

- **Travel and Exploration:**
    - Exploring travel opportunities, whether locally or internationally.
    - Group travel experiences that provide opportunities for social interactions.

7.9 Overcoming Barriers to Social Engagement

Seniors may encounter barriers to social engagement, ranging from mobility challenges to feelings of loneliness. This section addresses common barriers and provides practical strategies for overcoming them, emphasizing the importance of proactive approaches.

- **Mobility Challenges:**
    - Accessible transportation options and community initiatives that address mobility issues.
    - Creating environments that accommodate various mobility levels.

- **Technological Barriers:**
    - Addressing potential challenges seniors may face in adopting technology for social interactions.
    - Providing support and training to enhance digital literacy.

- **Language and Cultural Sensitivity:**

- Strategies for creating inclusive environments that respect diverse linguistic and cultural backgrounds.
- Cultivating awareness and understanding of cultural differences to foster a welcoming atmosphere.

7.10 Nurturing Lifelong Learning and Intellectual Engagement

Intellectual engagement contributes to the vitality of seniors, promoting ongoing learning and mental stimulation. This section explores avenues for intellectual enrichment and lifelong learning.

- **Educational Programs for Seniors:**
    - Accessing educational programs specifically designed for seniors, including lectures, workshops, and courses.
    - The benefits of continued learning in maintaining cognitive function.

- **Book Clubs and Discussion Groups:**
    - Joining book clubs or discussion groups that provide opportunities for intellectual exchange.
    - The role of shared reading experiences in fostering social connections.

- **Creative Pursuits:**
    - Engaging in creative pursuits such as writing, painting, or music.
    - Collaborative projects that encourage seniors to express themselves and share their creations.

7.11 Establishing Supportive Social Networks in Residential Settings

For seniors residing in communal settings, the chapter explores the importance of creating supportive social networks within these environments. It addresses communal living challenges and provides strategies for establishing inclusive and vibrant communities.

- **Communal Spaces and Activities:**
    - Designing communal spaces that facilitate social interactions among residents.
    - Organizing diverse activities to cater to different interests and preferences.

- **Residents' Associations:**
    - The role of residents' associations in fostering community engagement and addressing shared concerns.
    - Encouraging active participation in residents' meetings and decision-making processes.

- **Inclusive Events and Celebrations:**
    - Planning events and celebrations that celebrate diversity and inclusivity.
    - The impact of shared experiences in building a sense of community.

7.12 Recognizing the Individuality of Social Preferences

This section emphasizes the importance of recognizing and respecting the individuality of seniors' social preferences. It encourages a person-centered approach, acknowledging that social needs and preferences vary widely among older individuals.

- **Tailoring Social Activities to Preferences:**
    - Customizing social activities to align with individual interests and preferences.
    - Offering a variety of options to cater to diverse social needs.

- **Respecting Introversion and Extroversion:**
    - Acknowledging and accommodating

differences in social preferences, whether introverted or extroverted.

- Providing opportunities for both group interactions and solitary activities.

- **Effective Communication Strategies:**
    - Ensuring open communication channels for expressing social preferences.
    - Creating environments where seniors feel comfortable articulating their desires and boundaries.

7.13 Addressing Mental Health in Social Environments

Mental health considerations play a significant role in creating supportive social environments for seniors. This section explores strategies for recognizing and addressing mental health challenges, emphasizing the importance of a holistic approach.

- **Mental Health Awareness Programs:**
    - Implementing programs that raise awareness about mental health and reduce stigma.
    - Encouraging open conversations about mental well-being.

- **Access to Mental Health Services:**
    - Ensuring accessibility to mental health services within residential settings.
    - Collaboration with mental health professionals to provide on-site support.

- **Creating a Positive and Inclusive Atmosphere:**
    - Strategies for fostering positive and inclusive atmospheres that contribute to mental well-being.
    - The role of collective efforts in creating environments that prioritize mental health.

7.14 Evaluating and Adapting Social Programs

Evaluating the effectiveness of social programs is crucial for continuously enhancing the quality of life for seniors. This section provides guidance on assessing the impact of social initiatives and making adaptations based on feedback and evolving needs.

- **Collecting Resident Feedback:**
    - Implementing regular surveys and feedback mechanisms to gather input from seniors.
    - Actively seeking suggestions for improvements and new initiatives.

- **Flexibility in Program Design:**
    - Designing social programs with flexibility to accommodate changing preferences and demographics.
    - The role of iterative planning and adaptability in enhancing program effectiveness.

- **Measuring Social Impact:**
    - Developing metrics to measure the social impact of programs on seniors' well-being.
    - Utilizing data and feedback to make informed decisions about program modifications.

7.15 Encouraging Interconnectedness Beyond Residential Settings

While communal living provides a built-in social environment, seniors should also be encouraged to maintain connections beyond residential settings. This section explores ways to foster interconnectedness with the broader community.

- **Community Outreach Initiatives:**
    - Engaging in community outreach activities to connect with neighbors and local organizations.

- Collaborative efforts that benefit both seniors and the wider community.
- **Interactions with Local Businesses:**
    - Encouraging partnerships with local businesses to create opportunities for social interactions.
    - The role of businesses in supporting and catering to the needs of seniors.
- **Participation in Community Events:**
    - Actively participating in community events, festivals, and initiatives.
    - The reciprocal benefits of seniors contributing to and engaging with the larger community.

7.16 Navigating Changes and Transitions in Social Environments

This section addresses the challenges associated with changes in social environments, including transitions to new living arrangements or adjustments due to health conditions. It provides guidance on coping strategies and maintaining social well-being during periods of change.

- **Support Systems During Transitions:**
    - The importance of supportive networks during transitions, including moves to new residences or changes in health status.
    - Engaging in open communication with caregivers, family, and friends.
- **Adapting Social Programs:**
    - Strategies for adapting social programs to accommodate changing needs and circumstances.
    - Ensuring continuity in social support during transitions.

- **Embracing New Opportunities:**
    - Encouraging seniors to view changes as opportunities for new social connections and experiences.
    - The potential for personal growth and resilience during times of transition.

7.17 The Role of Caregivers and Family in Social Support

Caregivers and family members play a vital role in providing social support for seniors. This section explores the responsibilities of caregivers in facilitating and enhancing social connections, considering both formal and informal caregiving relationships.

- **Facilitating Social Activities:**
    - Caregiver involvement in organizing and facilitating social activities.
    - Collaborative efforts between caregivers and seniors in planning events and outings.

- **Open Communication with Caregivers:**
    - The importance of transparent communication between seniors and caregivers regarding social preferences and needs.
    - Regular discussions to address any challenges or concerns related to social well-being.

- **Respite Care to Support Social Engagement:**
    - Utilizing respite care services to provide caregivers with time for self-care and social activities.
    - The positive impact of respite care on the overall well-being of both seniors and caregivers.

7.18 Cultural Competence in Social Programming

Cultural competence is essential in creating social programs that cater to the diverse needs and preferences of seniors from various cultural backgrounds. This section explores the importance of cultural sensitivity and strategies for ensuring inclusivity in social programming.

- **Understanding Cultural Diversity:**
    - Acknowledging and appreciating the cultural diversity among seniors.
    - Creating programs that respect and celebrate various cultural traditions and practices.

- **Multilingual Communication:**
    - The role of multilingual communication in ensuring that all seniors can participate and engage comfortably.
    - Providing translation services or materials in multiple languages.

- **Celebrating Cultural Festivals and Events:**
    - Incorporating cultural celebrations and events into social programs.
    - The positive impact of shared cultural experiences in fostering a sense of community.

7.19 Collaborations with Local Organizations and Initiatives

Collaborations with local organizations, nonprofits, and community initiatives can significantly enhance the social well-being of seniors. This section explores the benefits of partnerships and offers guidance on establishing and maintaining fruitful collaborations.

- **Networking with Local Groups:**
    - Establishing connections with local senior centers, community groups, and organizations.
    - Collaborative efforts in planning joint events and initiatives.

- **Participating in Community Initiatives:**

- Engaging in broader community initiatives that address social issues and enhance the overall well-being of seniors.
- The reciprocal benefits of seniors contributing to and being involved in community projects.

- **Access to External Resources:**
  - Tapping into external resources provided by local organizations, such as educational programs, recreational opportunities, and support services.
  - The role of local initiatives in complementing and expanding social programs within residential settings.

7.20 Ensuring Dignity and Respect in Social Interactions

Dignity and respect are foundational elements in creating a supportive social environment for seniors. This section emphasizes the importance of fostering an atmosphere where all individuals are treated with dignity, regardless of age or health status.

- **Promoting Inclusive Language:**
  - Encouraging the use of inclusive language that respects seniors' autonomy and individuality.
  - Addressing ageist stereotypes and language that may perpetuate negative perceptions.

- **Creating Safe Spaces:**
  - Establishing environments where seniors feel safe expressing themselves and engaging in social interactions.
  - The impact of feeling respected and valued on overall well-being.

- **Zero Tolerance for Ageism:**
  - Advocating for a zero-tolerance policy against

ageism in social programs and interactions.

- Promoting education and awareness to eliminate age-based discrimination.

7.21 Evaluating Social Impact on Overall Well-being

This section explores the interconnectedness between social engagement and overall well-being for seniors. It delves into methodologies for evaluating the social impact on physical, mental, and emotional health, emphasizing the holistic nature of well-being.

- **Measuring Physical Health Outcomes:**
  - Evaluating physical health indicators influenced by social engagement, such as mobility, cardiovascular health, and sleep patterns.
  - Collaborating with healthcare professionals to assess the impact of social activities on specific health goals.

- **Assessing Emotional Well-being:**
  - Utilizing self-assessment tools and surveys to gauge emotional well-being in relation to social interactions.
  - The role of regular check-ins and open communication in understanding emotional health.

- **Cognitive Function and Social Stimulation:**
  - Monitoring cognitive function and memory recall in connection with social engagement.
  - Incorporating cognitive assessments to understand the cognitive benefits of social activities.

7.22 Adapting to Changing Social Needs

Seniors' social needs evolve over time, influenced by factors such as health changes, life events, and personal preferences. This section provides insights into adapting social programs and support systems to meet changing needs and ensure continued social well-being.

- **Regular Social Assessments:**
  - Implementing regular assessments to understand evolving social needs.
  - The importance of open communication with seniors to gather insights into their changing preferences.

- **Flexible Program Design:**
  - Designing social programs with flexibility to accommodate varying levels of participation and preferences.
  - The role of adaptability in ensuring that programs remain relevant and engaging.

- **Collaborative Decision-Making:**
  - Involving seniors in decision-making processes related to social programming.
  - Creating platforms for feedback and suggestions to shape the direction of social initiatives.

7.23 Celebrating Milestones and Achievements

This section highlights the significance of celebrating milestones and achievements within social programs. Recognizing individual and collective accomplishments contributes to a positive and supportive social environment.

- **Acknowledging Personal Milestones:**
  - Celebrating individual achievements, whether big or small.

- Creating a culture of recognition and appreciation within social groups.
- **Communal Celebrations:**
  - Organizing communal celebrations for achievements within the broader community.
  - The positive impact of shared celebrations in fostering a sense of unity.
- **Building a Culture of Encouragement:**
  - Encouraging a supportive culture where seniors uplift and celebrate each other.
  - The reciprocal benefits of contributing to a positive and encouraging social atmosphere.

7.24 Future Trends in Senior Social Engagement

The chapter concludes by exploring emerging trends in senior social engagement. It discusses the potential impact of technological advancements, changes in societal attitudes, and evolving preferences among seniors. Anticipating future trends allows for proactive adaptation and enhancement of social programs.

- **Integration of Virtual Reality:**
  - The potential role of virtual reality in creating immersive and interactive social experiences for seniors.
  - Exploring virtual travel, cultural events, and collaborative activities in a virtual space.
- **Enhanced Accessibility Through Technology:**
  - Advancements in technology to enhance accessibility for seniors with diverse abilities.
  - The integration of voice-activated devices, smart home features, and other innovations in social programs.

- **Holistic Wellness Integration:**
    - Future trends in integrating social engagement with holistic wellness programs.
    - The intersection of physical, mental, and emotional well-being in comprehensive social initiatives.

- **Personalized Social Experiences:**
    - The rise of personalized social experiences tailored to individual preferences and interests.
    - Leveraging technology and data to create customized social programs that resonate with seniors.

- **Community-Led Initiatives:**
    - The potential growth of grassroots community-led initiatives in promoting senior social engagement.
    - Empowering seniors to take active roles in shaping their social environments and programs.

In conclusion, fostering a supportive social environment for seniors is a dynamic and multifaceted endeavor. By understanding the unique needs, preferences, and challenges faced by older individuals, communities, caregivers, and organizations can collaborate to create vibrant, inclusive, and enriching social programs that contribute to the overall well-being of seniors.

CHAPTER 8: NUTRITION AND HEALTH FOR SENIOR WELL-BEING

Maintaining optimal health is crucial for seniors to lead fulfilling and independent lives. Nutrition plays a pivotal role in promoting well-being, supporting immune function, and preventing chronic conditions. This chapter delves into the unique nutritional needs of seniors, strategies for maintaining a healthy diet, and the integration of nutrition into comprehensive health plans.

8.1 Understanding the Changing Nutritional Needs of Seniors

As individuals age, their bodies undergo physiological changes that can impact nutritional requirements. This section explores the specific nutritional needs of seniors, addressing factors such as metabolism, digestion, and nutrient absorption.

- **Metabolic Changes:**
    - Understanding the gradual decline in metabolic rate and its impact on calorie needs.
    - Strategies for adjusting dietary habits to accommodate metabolic changes without compromising nutrition.

- **Digestive System Changes:**
    - Exploring changes in the digestive system, including reduced stomach acid production and slower digestion.
    - Dietary modifications to enhance nutrient absorption and alleviate digestive discomfort.

- **Nutrient Absorption Challenges:**
    - Recognizing potential challenges in absorbing

certain nutrients, such as vitamin B12 and calcium.

- Dietary sources and supplements to address specific nutrient deficiencies common in seniors.

8.2 The Role of Nutrition in Preventing Chronic Conditions

Seniors face an increased risk of developing chronic conditions, making preventive nutrition a crucial aspect of their health. This section examines the links between nutrition and common age-related health concerns, including heart disease, osteoporosis, and cognitive decline.

- **Heart Health and Nutrition:**
    - Exploring dietary strategies to promote cardiovascular health, including the consumption of heart-healthy fats, fiber, and antioxidants.
    - The role of nutrient-dense foods in lowering cholesterol levels and maintaining blood pressure.

- **Bone Health and Osteoporosis Prevention:**
    - The significance of calcium and vitamin D in maintaining bone density.
    - Dietary sources and supplementation recommendations for preventing osteoporosis.

- **Cognitive Health and Brain Function:**
    - Examining the impact of nutrition on cognitive function and reducing the risk of cognitive decline.
    - Foods rich in antioxidants, omega-3 fatty acids, and other brain-supportive nutrients.

8.3 Strategies for Achieving a Balanced and Nutrient-Rich Diet

This section provides practical strategies for seniors to achieve a balanced and nutrient-rich diet. It explores dietary guidelines, meal planning, and the incorporation of a variety of foods to meet essential nutritional needs.

- **Dietary Guidelines for Seniors:**
  - Overview of dietary guidelines tailored to the needs of seniors, including recommended servings of fruits, vegetables, whole grains, and lean proteins.
  - The importance of maintaining hydration and limiting sodium intake.

- **Meal Planning for Seniors:**
  - Strategies for effective meal planning that considers individual preferences, dietary restrictions, and nutritional requirements.
  - Weekly meal preparation and batch cooking for convenience and nutritional consistency.

- **Incorporating Varied Food Groups:**
  - The importance of including a diverse range of foods to ensure a broad spectrum of nutrients.
  - Creative approaches to incorporating fruits, vegetables, proteins, and whole grains into daily meals.

8.4 Addressing Common Nutritional Challenges in Seniors

Seniors may encounter specific challenges related to nutrition, from decreased appetite to dental issues. This section identifies common hurdles and provides solutions to ensure adequate nutrition for overall health and well-being.

- **Decreased Appetite:**
  - Understanding factors that contribute to a decreased appetite in seniors, such as changes

in taste and smell.

- Strategies to stimulate appetite, including flavorful cooking techniques and smaller, more frequent meals.

- **Dental Health Considerations:**
  - The impact of dental issues on food choices and dietary habits.

  - Soft and easy-to-chew food options, as well as dental hygiene practices to support oral health.

- **Digestive Issues:**
  - Addressing common digestive issues in seniors, such as constipation and indigestion.

  - Dietary fiber recommendations and hydration strategies to promote healthy digestion.

8.5 Hydration and Its Importance for Senior Health

Proper hydration is integral to overall health, yet seniors may be at an increased risk of dehydration. This section explores the significance of hydration for seniors, methods to ensure adequate fluid intake, and the role of various beverages in supporting health.

- **Dehydration Risks in Seniors:**
  - Identifying factors that contribute to dehydration in seniors, including reduced thirst sensation and medication side effects.

  - The impact of dehydration on health, including kidney function, cognitive performance, and temperature regulation.

- **Ensuring Adequate Fluid Intake:**
  - Strategies for seniors to maintain proper hydration levels, including setting regular reminders and incorporating hydrating foods.

- The role of water, herbal teas, and hydrating foods in supporting overall hydration.
- **Healthful Beverage Choices:**
  - Exploring healthful beverage options beyond water, including herbal teas, infused water, and low-sugar fruit juices.
  - Limiting the consumption of sugary and caffeinated beverages to promote optimal hydration.

8.6 Weight Management and Healthy Eating Habits

Maintaining a healthy weight is crucial for seniors, and this section explores the principles of weight management and the cultivation of positive eating habits. It addresses factors such as portion control, mindful eating, and the role of regular physical activity in weight maintenance.

- **Portion Control Strategies:**
  - Guidelines for portion control to prevent overeating and support weight management.
  - The importance of listening to hunger and fullness cues.

- **Mindful Eating Practices:**
  - Exploring mindful eating as a strategy to enhance the enjoyment of meals and promote healthier food choices.
  - Techniques such as savoring flavors, paying attention to hunger signals, and avoiding distractions during meals.

- **Incorporating Physical Activity:**
  - The synergistic relationship between nutrition and physical activity for weight management.
  - Tailoring dietary choices to support energy levels and nutritional needs for seniors engaged

in regular physical activity.

8.7 Dietary Considerations for Common Health Conditions

Seniors often manage chronic health conditions, and dietary choices can significantly impact the management of these conditions. This section provides insights into dietary considerations for conditions such as diabetes, hypertension, and gastrointestinal issues.

- **Managing Diabetes through Diet:**
    - The role of carbohydrate control, fiber intake, and balanced meals in diabetes management.
    - Strategies for monitoring blood sugar levels through dietary choices.

- **Dietary Approaches for Hypertension:**
    - Exploring the impact of sodium, potassium, and heart-healthy fats on blood pressure.
    - Dietary modifications to support hypertension management.

- **Promoting Gastrointestinal Health:**
    - Dietary recommendations for seniors dealing with gastrointestinal conditions, such as irritable bowel syndrome (IBS) or constipation.
    - The role of fiber, hydration, and specific food choices in maintaining gastrointestinal well-being.

8.8 Nutritional Supplements for Seniors

While a well-balanced diet is ideal, nutritional supplements can be valuable for seniors to address specific deficiencies or challenges. This section explores the role of supplements, including vitamins, minerals, and other essential nutrients, in supporting senior health.

- **Common Nutritional Deficiencies in Seniors:**
  - Identifying prevalent deficiencies in nutrients such as vitamin D, vitamin B12, calcium, and omega-3 fatty acids.
  - The impact of deficiencies on health and well-being.

- **Considerations for Supplement Use:**
  - Guidelines for incorporating nutritional supplements, including dosage recommendations and potential interactions with medications.
  - The importance of consulting healthcare professionals before initiating supplement regimens.

- **Individualized Supplement Plans:**
  - Tailoring supplement plans based on individual nutritional needs and health conditions.
  - Regular assessment of nutrient levels to adjust supplement regimens as necessary.

8.9 Culinary Exploration and Enjoyable Eating Experiences

Seniors can enhance their nutritional intake and overall well-being by embracing culinary exploration and enjoying diverse eating experiences. This section encourages seniors to explore new foods, cuisines, and cooking techniques to make the dining experience more enjoyable.

- **Exploring Culinary Diversity:**
  - Encouraging seniors to try new fruits, vegetables, whole grains, and ethnic cuisines.
  - The nutritional benefits and sensory pleasures of embracing a varied and colorful diet.

- **Cooking Classes and Social Culinary Events:**
  - Participating in cooking classes or social

culinary events to enhance culinary skills and share enjoyable experiences with peers.

- The role of communal cooking and shared meals in fostering social connections.

- **Gardening and Farm-to-Table Experiences:**
    - The benefits of gardening for seniors, including access to fresh produce and the joy of cultivating one's food.

    - Participating in farm-to-table experiences and farmers' markets to connect with locally sourced, seasonal foods.

8.10 Cultural and Personalized Dietary Preferences

Seniors often have unique cultural and personalized dietary preferences that contribute to their sense of identity and well-being. This section explores the importance of respecting and incorporating these preferences into nutritional plans.

- **Cultural Influences on Dietary Choices:**
    - Recognizing the impact of cultural background on dietary preferences and habits.

    - Strategies for integrating cultural traditions into meal planning and nutritional support.

- **Respecting Individual Dietary Preferences:**
    - Tailoring nutritional advice to align with individual tastes, dietary restrictions, and ethical choices.

    - The importance of creating flexible dietary plans that accommodate diverse preferences.

- **Celebrating Food as a Source of Joy and Connection:**
    - Fostering a positive and celebratory attitude towards food as a source of joy and connection.

    - Incorporating favorite dishes and nostalgic

foods into regular meals for emotional well-being.

8.11 The Role of Caregivers and Family in Nutritional Support

Caregivers and family members play a significant role in supporting seniors' nutritional well-being. This section explores the responsibilities of caregivers in meal preparation, nutritional monitoring, and fostering a positive eating environment.

- **Collaborative Meal Planning:**
    - Collaborating with seniors in meal planning to incorporate their preferences and nutritional needs.
    - The positive impact of involving seniors in grocery shopping and meal preparation.

- **Ensuring Nutritional Support during Health Challenges:**
    - The role of caregivers in providing nutritional support during periods of illness, recovery, or changes in health status.
    - Collaborative efforts with healthcare professionals to address nutritional challenges.

- **Creating Enjoyable Dining Environments:**
    - Fostering enjoyable dining experiences by creating pleasant and relaxed mealtime environments.
    - Strategies for enhancing social connections during meals, such as family gatherings or shared dining with peers.

8.12 Sustainable and Ethical Eating Practices

As awareness of environmental and ethical considerations grows, seniors may express interest in sustainable and ethical eating practices. This section explores the connection between nutrition, sustainability, and ethical food choices.

- **Choosing Sustainable and Local Foods:**
    - The environmental impact of food choices and the benefits of choosing locally sourced, seasonal produce.
    - Participating in sustainable agriculture initiatives and supporting local farmers.
- **Ethical Considerations in Food Production:**
    - Exploring ethical considerations related to food production, including animal welfare and fair labor practices.
    - Strategies for making ethically informed choices when purchasing food products.
- **Reducing Food Waste:**
    - The impact of food waste on the environment and strategies for minimizing waste in daily meals.
    - Creative approaches to repurposing leftovers and utilizing ingredients efficiently.

8.13 Continuous Monitoring and Adjustments to Nutritional Plans

Seniors' nutritional needs can change over time due to factors such as health conditions, medications, and lifestyle adjustments. This section emphasizes the importance of continuous monitoring and making necessary adjustments to nutritional plans.

- **Regular Health Assessments:**
    - The role of regular health assessments in identifying changes in nutritional needs.
    - Collaborating with healthcare professionals to address evolving health conditions and adjust dietary recommendations.
- **Communication with Healthcare Providers:**

- Encouraging open communication between seniors, caregivers, and healthcare providers regarding dietary concerns and challenges.
- The potential role of registered dietitians in providing specialized nutritional guidance.

- **Adapting to Lifestyle Changes:**
    - Strategies for adapting nutritional plans to align with lifestyle changes, such as transitions to different living arrangements or alterations in daily routines.
    - Flexibility in dietary recommendations to accommodate evolving preferences and circumstances.

8.14 Utilizing Technology for Nutritional Support

Technology can play a valuable role in supporting seniors' nutritional well-being. This section explores the use of apps, online resources, and smart devices to enhance nutritional knowledge, monitor dietary habits, and facilitate convenient access to nutritional information.

- **Nutrition Apps and Trackers:**
    - The benefits of using nutrition apps to track dietary intake, set nutritional goals, and receive personalized recommendations.
    - Exploring user-friendly apps that cater to seniors' specific needs and preferences.

- **Online Nutrition Resources:**
    - Accessing reliable online resources for nutritional information, recipes, and meal planning guidance.
    - The role of reputable websites and digital platforms in providing up-to-date nutritional advice.

- **Smart Kitchen Appliances:**
    - The potential advantages of incorporating smart kitchen appliances, such as smart scales or voice-activated assistants, to enhance the cooking and meal preparation process.
    - Technological innovations that contribute to a more streamlined and efficient kitchen experience.

8.15 Promoting Well-being Through Culinary and Nutritional Education

Culinary and nutritional education can empower seniors to make informed food choices, enhance their cooking skills, and derive greater enjoyment from their meals. This section explores the benefits of educational initiatives focused on nutrition and culinary practices.

- **Cooking Classes for Seniors:**
    - The positive impact of cooking classes tailored to seniors' needs, providing hands-on experience and practical tips.
    - Collaborations with local chefs or nutritionists to offer engaging and informative classes.

- **Nutritional Workshops and Seminars:**
    - Hosting nutritional workshops and seminars to provide seniors with the latest information on dietary trends, superfoods, and personalized nutrition.
    - Encouraging active participation and discussions to address individual concerns and questions.

- **Community Gardens and Nutrition Gardens:**
    - Establishing community gardens or nutrition gardens to promote hands-on involvement in

growing and harvesting nutritious produce.

- The educational benefits of connecting seniors with the food production process.

8.16 Evaluating Nutritional Impact on Overall Well-being

This section explores the interconnectedness between nutritional choices and overall well-being for seniors. It delves into methodologies for evaluating the impact of nutrition on physical health, cognitive function, emotional well-being, and social interactions.

- **Physical Health Indicators:**
  - Monitoring physical health indicators influenced by nutrition, such as energy levels, weight management, and chronic disease management.
  - The role of regular health check-ups in assessing the physical impact of nutrition.

- **Cognitive Function and Nutrition:**
  - Examining the relationship between nutritional choices and cognitive function.
  - The potential cognitive benefits of a well-balanced diet rich in antioxidants and omega-3 fatty acids.

- **Emotional and Social Aspects of Nutrition:**
  - Considering the emotional and social aspects of nutrition, including the joy derived from shared meals and culinary experiences.
  - Evaluating the impact of nutrition on mental well-being and social interactions.

8.17 Adapting Nutritional Plans to Changing Health Needs

Seniors may experience changes in health needs that require adjustments to their nutritional plans. This section provides guidance on adapting nutritional strategies to accommodate evolving health conditions and maintaining overall well-being.

- **Dietary Modifications for Health Conditions:**
    - Tailoring nutritional plans to address specific health conditions, such as diabetes, heart disease, or dietary restrictions.
    - Collaborating with healthcare professionals to integrate nutritional support into overall health management.

- **Nutritional Support during Recovery:**
    - Strategies for providing nutritional support during periods of recovery from surgery, illness, or medical treatments.
    - The role of nutrient-dense foods in supporting the healing process.

- **Holistic Approaches to Nutritional Well-being:**
    - The importance of adopting holistic approaches to nutritional well-being that consider physical, mental, and emotional health.
    - Collaborating with multidisciplinary healthcare teams to integrate nutritional support into comprehensive care plans.

8.18 Supporting Seniors in Making Informed Nutritional Choices

Empowering seniors to make informed nutritional choices is a key aspect of promoting their overall well-being. This section explores educational initiatives, resources, and strategies for fostering nutritional literacy and autonomy.

- **Accessible Nutritional Information:**
    - Ensuring that nutritional information is presented in an accessible and comprehensible manner for seniors.

- The role of clear labeling and easy-to-understand nutritional facts on food packaging.

- **Nutritional Counseling Services:**
  - The benefits of offering nutritional counseling services to seniors, providing personalized guidance and support.

  - Collaborating with registered dietitians or nutritionists to address individual nutritional needs.

- **Encouraging Informed Decision-Making:**
  - Fostering an environment where seniors feel empowered to make informed decisions about their nutritional choices.

  - Encouraging questions, discussions, and shared decision-making in the realm of nutrition.

8.19 Collaboration with Healthcare Providers for Holistic Care

Collaboration between nutrition professionals and healthcare providers is essential for delivering holistic care to seniors. This section explores the integration of nutritional support into healthcare plans and the benefits of interdisciplinary collaboration.

- **Incorporating Nutrition into Healthcare Plans:**
  - Recognizing the importance of nutrition in overall healthcare plans for seniors.

  - Collaborative efforts between nutritionists, physicians, and other healthcare professionals to address comprehensive health needs.

- **Regular Communication between Care Teams:**
  - The value of regular communication between care teams to ensure that nutritional plans align with overall health goals.

  - Utilizing interdisciplinary meetings to discuss

individual cases and coordinate care.

- **Educating Healthcare Providers on Nutrition:**
    - Providing ongoing education for healthcare providers on the latest developments in nutritional science and guidelines.
    - Facilitating a shared understanding of the role of nutrition in promoting health and preventing chronic conditions.

8.20 Future Trends in Senior Nutrition

The chapter concludes by exploring emerging trends in senior nutrition. It considers the potential impact of technological advancements, personalized nutrition approaches, and evolving dietary preferences. Anticipating future trends allows for proactive adaptation and enhancement of nutritional programs.

- **Personalized Nutrition Plans:**
    - The potential rise of personalized nutrition plans tailored to individual health needs, genetic factors, and preferences.
    - Utilizing technology and data to create customized nutritional recommendations.

- **Integration of Culinary Medicine:**
    - The incorporation of culinary medicine principles into nutritional approaches, emphasizing the therapeutic aspects of food.
    - Collaborations between nutrition professionals and culinary experts to integrate culinary medicine into senior care.

- **Innovations in Nutritional Supplements:**
    - Advancements in the development of nutritional supplements, including tailored formulations and targeted delivery systems.
    - The potential role of cutting-edge supplements

in addressing specific health concerns in seniors.

- **Nutritional Interventions for Cognitive Health:**
  - Research and developments in nutritional interventions aimed at supporting cognitive health and preventing age-related cognitive decline.
  - The exploration of dietary patterns with neuroprotective effects.

- **Technological Support for Nutritional Monitoring:**
  - The integration of wearable devices and smart technology to monitor nutritional intake, hydration levels, and overall dietary patterns.
  - Real-time data collection to inform personalized nutritional recommendations.

In conclusion, prioritizing nutrition is fundamental to ensuring the well-being of seniors. By understanding their unique nutritional needs, addressing challenges, and embracing innovative approaches, communities, caregivers, and healthcare professionals can contribute to the holistic health and longevity of seniors.

CHAPTER 9: MENTAL AND EMOTIONAL WELL-BEING FOR SENIORS

Promoting mental and emotional well-being is essential for seniors to lead fulfilling lives as they navigate the challenges and opportunities that come with aging. This chapter delves into the multifaceted aspects of mental and emotional health, exploring strategies for fostering resilience, maintaining cognitive vitality, and nurturing positive social connections.

9.1 The Significance of Mental and Emotional Well-being

As individuals age, mental and emotional well-being become integral components of overall health. This section highlights the importance of addressing the unique challenges and opportunities related to seniors' mental and emotional health.

- **Holistic Approach to Well-being:**
    - Recognizing the interconnectedness of mental, emotional, and physical well-being in the context of seniors' health.
    - The impact of mental and emotional health on overall quality of life and longevity.

- **Common Mental and Emotional Challenges:**
    - Identifying prevalent challenges faced by seniors, including loneliness, depression, anxiety, and cognitive decline.
    - Strategies for early detection and intervention to address mental health concerns.

- **Positive Outcomes of Prioritizing Well-being:**
    - Exploring the positive outcomes of prioritizing

mental and emotional well-being, including enhanced resilience, cognitive vitality, and a sense of purpose.

- The role of a positive mindset in navigating life transitions and maintaining a fulfilling lifestyle.

9.2 Cognitive Vitality and Brain Health

Maintaining cognitive vitality is crucial for seniors to sustain independence and engage actively in daily life. This section explores strategies for preserving cognitive function, stimulating the brain, and addressing age-related cognitive changes.

- **Understanding Age-related Cognitive Changes:**
  - Exploring normal age-related cognitive changes, such as slower processing speed and mild memory lapses.
  - Distinguishing between typical aging and signs of cognitive disorders.

- **Stimulating Cognitive Engagement:**
  - The importance of ongoing cognitive stimulation through activities such as puzzles, games, and learning.
  - Incorporating diverse cognitive exercises to challenge different aspects of cognitive function.

- **Promoting Lifelong Learning:**
  - Encouraging seniors to embrace lifelong learning through educational courses, workshops, and hobbies.
  - The cognitive benefits of acquiring new skills and knowledge throughout life.

9.3 Strategies for Building Resilience

Resilience is a key component of mental and emotional well-being, enabling seniors to adapt to challenges and bounce back from adversity. This section explores practical strategies for cultivating resilience in the face of life's ups and downs.

- **Developing Coping Mechanisms:**
  - Identifying and developing effective coping mechanisms to navigate stress, loss, and life changes.
  - Encouraging the cultivation of adaptive coping strategies that align with individual preferences.

- **Mindfulness and Stress Reduction Techniques:**
  - The role of mindfulness practices, meditation, and relaxation techniques in reducing stress and promoting emotional resilience.
  - Incorporating mindfulness into daily routines for enhanced emotional well-being.

- **Cultivating Positive Self-talk:**
  - Recognizing the impact of self-talk on emotional resilience.
  - Strategies for fostering a positive and self-compassionate internal dialogue.

9.4 Nurturing Social Connections and Combating Loneliness

Social connections are vital for seniors' mental and emotional well-being, yet they may face challenges such as isolation and loneliness. This section explores the importance of social engagement and strategies for fostering meaningful connections.

- **Impact of Social Connections on Well-being:**
  - Highlighting the positive impact of social connections on mental and emotional health.

- The role of social support in mitigating feelings of loneliness and enhancing overall well-being.

- **Diverse Social Engagement Opportunities:**
  - Encouraging seniors to explore diverse social engagement opportunities, including community groups, clubs, and volunteering.
  - Tailoring social activities to individual interests and preferences.

- **Utilizing Technology for Social Connection:**
  - Exploring the benefits of technology in facilitating virtual social connections, especially for seniors with limited mobility.
  - The potential of video calls, social media, and online communities in reducing social isolation.

9.5 Emotional Expression and Artistic Outlets

Creative expression and artistic outlets provide avenues for seniors to explore and express their emotions, contributing to mental and emotional well-being. This section explores the therapeutic benefits of engaging in various forms of artistic expression.

- **Art Therapy and Creative Outlets:**
  - The therapeutic benefits of art therapy, music, dance, and other creative outlets for emotional expression.
  - Collaborative projects and group activities to enhance social connections through artistic endeavors.

- **Journaling and Reflective Practices:**
  - Encouraging seniors to engage in journaling and reflective practices as a means of processing emotions and documenting life experiences.

- The cathartic effect of written expression in promoting emotional well-being.

- **Participation in Artistic Communities:**
    - Joining artistic communities and groups to share experiences, collaborate on projects, and build a sense of belonging.

    - The positive impact of shared creative pursuits on mental and emotional health.

9.6 Emotional Regulation and Stress Management Techniques

Emotional regulation and stress management are integral components of maintaining mental and emotional well-being. This section explores techniques and practices that support seniors in managing stress and regulating their emotional responses.

- **Mind-Body Practices:**
    - The role of mind-body practices such as yoga, tai chi, and qigong in promoting emotional regulation and stress reduction.

    - Incorporating gentle and mindful movement into daily routines.

- **Breathing Exercises and Relaxation Techniques:**
    - Teaching seniors breathing exercises and relaxation techniques to manage stress and anxiety.

    - The accessibility and effectiveness of simple techniques for immediate stress relief.

- **Cognitive Behavioral Strategies:**
    - Introducing cognitive-behavioral strategies to identify and challenge negative thought patterns.

    - The empowering effect of cognitive restructuring in promoting a positive mindset.

9.7 Addressing Depression and Anxiety in Seniors

Depression and anxiety can significantly impact the mental and emotional well-being of seniors. This section explores the identification of symptoms, intervention strategies, and the role of professional support in addressing these mental health concerns.

- **Recognizing Signs and Symptoms:**
  - Providing information on common signs and symptoms of depression and anxiety in seniors.
  - The importance of early detection and seeking professional help.

- **Therapeutic Interventions:**
  - Exploring therapeutic interventions, including counseling and psychotherapy, to address underlying emotional challenges.
  - The role of evidence-based therapeutic modalities in promoting mental health.

- **Collaboration with Healthcare Providers:**
  - The importance of collaborative efforts between mental health professionals and healthcare providers in developing comprehensive care plans.
  - Addressing the stigma associated with seeking mental health support in the senior population.

9.8 Supporting Seniors with Cognitive Disorders

Seniors dealing with cognitive disorders, such as Alzheimer's disease and dementia, require specialized support to maintain their mental and emotional well-being. This section addresses strategies for providing compassionate care and enhancing the quality of life for seniors with cognitive disorders.

- **Person-Centered Care Approaches:**
  - Adopting person-centered care approaches that prioritize the individual preferences, routines, and memories of seniors with cognitive disorders.
  - The positive impact of personalized and empathetic care on emotional well-being.

- **Engaging Memory-enhancing Activities:**
  - Incorporating memory-enhancing activities and cognitive stimulation to support seniors with cognitive disorders.
  - Creating a supportive environment that encourages engagement and minimizes frustration.

- **Family and Caregiver Support:**
  - Providing resources and support for family members and caregivers of seniors with cognitive disorders.
  - The importance of self-care for caregivers in maintaining their own mental and emotional well-being.

9.9 Meaningful End-of-life Conversations and Planning

End-of-life conversations and planning are integral aspects of comprehensive care for seniors. This section explores the importance of addressing end-of-life preferences, fostering a sense of purpose, and supporting seniors in navigating this significant aspect of their lives.

- **Advance Care Planning:**
  - Encouraging seniors to engage in advance care planning, including discussions on healthcare preferences, living arrangements, and end-of-life decisions.

- The role of legal documents such as advance directives and durable power of attorney in ensuring their wishes are honored.

- **Exploring Life's Purpose and Legacy:**
    - Facilitating conversations on life's purpose, values, and the creation of a meaningful legacy.

    - Supporting seniors in reflecting on and sharing their life stories with loved ones.

- **Spiritual and Existential Exploration:**
    - Recognizing the spiritual and existential dimensions of well-being in the context of end-of-life discussions.

    - Providing opportunities for seniors to explore and express their beliefs, fears, and hopes regarding the end of life.

9.10 Integrating Technology for Cognitive and Emotional Support

Technology can play a significant role in providing cognitive and emotional support for seniors. This section explores the utilization of apps, virtual reality, and other technological innovations to enhance mental and emotional well-being.

- **Cognitive Training Apps:**
    - The benefits of cognitive training apps designed to stimulate various cognitive functions, memory, and problem-solving skills.

    - Customizing app usage based on individual interests and preferences.

- **Virtual Reality for Therapeutic Purposes:**
    - Exploring the therapeutic applications of virtual reality in addressing anxiety, depression, and providing immersive experiences for seniors.

- Collaborations with healthcare professionals to integrate virtual reality into mental health interventions.

- **Social Media and Online Support Groups:**
  - The potential positive impact of social media and online support groups in reducing social isolation and facilitating connections among seniors.

  - Encouraging safe and meaningful online interactions for emotional support.

9.11 Promoting Sleep Hygiene and Its Impact on Mental Well-being

Quality sleep is fundamental to mental and emotional well-being, yet seniors may face challenges in maintaining healthy sleep patterns. This section explores the importance of sleep hygiene and strategies for promoting restful sleep.

- **Understanding Age-related Sleep Changes:**
  - Identifying age-related changes in sleep patterns and the impact on mental health.

  - Distinguishing between normal sleep changes and potential sleep disorders.

- **Promoting Sleep Hygiene Practices:**
  - Providing guidelines for promoting good sleep hygiene, including consistent sleep schedules, a comfortable sleep environment, and relaxation techniques.

  - Addressing common sleep disruptions and fostering healthy bedtime routines.

- **Addressing Sleep Disorders:**
  - Recognizing signs of sleep disorders in seniors, such as insomnia or sleep apnea.

  - Collaboration with healthcare providers to

diagnose and address sleep disorders for improved mental and emotional well-being.

9.12 Physical Activity and Its Impact on Mental Health

Physical activity is closely linked to mental well-being, and seniors can benefit from regular exercise to support their emotional health. This section explores the positive impact of physical activity on mental health and strategies for incorporating exercise into daily routines.

- **The Mind-Body Connection:**
    - Understanding the interconnectedness of physical activity and mental health.
    - The release of endorphins and other neurotransmitters during exercise that contribute to improved mood.

- **Tailoring Exercise Routines for Seniors:**
    - Providing guidance on age-appropriate and enjoyable exercise routines for seniors.
    - The importance of incorporating a variety of activities, including aerobic exercise, strength training, and flexibility exercises.

- **Socially Engaging Physical Activities:**
    - Encouraging physically active pursuits that also foster social connections, such as group walks, dancing, or team sports.
    - The dual benefit of social engagement and physical activity in promoting mental well-being.

9.13 Exploring Nature and Outdoor Activities

Nature and outdoor activities have therapeutic benefits for mental and emotional well-being. This section delves into the positive impact of nature on seniors' mental health and strategies for incorporating outdoor activities into their lifestyles.

- **Nature's Therapeutic Effects:**
    - Exploring the calming and rejuvenating effects of nature on mental health.
    - The concept of ecotherapy and the potential benefits of spending time in natural settings.

- **Outdoor Activities for Seniors:**
    - Encouraging seniors to engage in outdoor activities such as walking, gardening, birdwatching, or picnics.
    - The importance of exposure to natural light and fresh air for improved mood and cognitive function.

- **Community Green Spaces and Initiatives:**
    - Advocating for the creation and maintenance of community green spaces that facilitate outdoor activities for seniors.
    - Collaborations with local initiatives to promote nature-based interventions for mental and emotional well-being.

9.14 Volunteerism and Purposeful Engagement

Engaging in volunteer activities and finding a sense of purpose contribute significantly to seniors' mental and emotional well-being. This section explores the positive impact of volunteerism and strategies for seniors to discover purposeful engagement.

- **Benefits of Volunteerism:**
    - Highlighting the physical, mental, and emotional benefits of volunteering for seniors.
    - The sense of purpose and fulfillment derived from contributing to the community.

- **Identifying Personal Interests and Passions:**
    - Encouraging seniors to explore and identify personal interests, hobbies, and passions.
    - The positive impact of pursuing meaningful activities that align with individual values.

- **Connecting Seniors with Volunteer Opportunities:**
    - Providing resources and support to connect seniors with volunteer opportunities in their communities.
    - Tailoring volunteer roles to match seniors' skills, interests, and physical abilities.

9.15 Encouraging Lifelong Learning and Intellectual Stimulation

Intellectual stimulation and lifelong learning are key components of cognitive vitality and mental well-being. This section explores strategies for seniors to engage in continuous learning and intellectual pursuits.

- **Educational Programs and Courses:**
    - The availability of educational programs, courses, and workshops for seniors.
    - Exploring opportunities for lifelong learning through local community colleges, online platforms, and senior centers.

- **Book Clubs and Discussion Groups:**
    - The social and intellectual benefits of participating in book clubs or discussion groups.
    - Creating spaces for seniors to share thoughts, ideas, and engage in stimulating conversations.

- **Creative Writing and Memory Exercises:**
    - Incorporating creative writing exercises, memory games, and puzzles to stimulate

cognitive function.

- The therapeutic and enjoyable aspects of engaging in creative and intellectual pursuits.

9.16 Fostering Intergenerational Connections

Interactions with younger generations bring joy, purpose, and a sense of connection to seniors. This section explores the positive impact of intergenerational relationships and strategies for fostering meaningful connections between seniors and younger individuals.

- **Benefits of Intergenerational Connections:**
  - Recognizing the reciprocal benefits for both seniors and younger generations in intergenerational interactions.
  - The exchange of wisdom, experiences, and the creation of lasting bonds.

- **Intergenerational Programs and Activities:**
  - The implementation of intergenerational programs, such as mentorship initiatives, joint activities, and collaborative projects.
  - Creating opportunities for shared experiences that bridge generational gaps.

- **Family Involvement and Communication:**
  - Encouraging open communication and involvement of family members in facilitating intergenerational connections.
  - The role of family gatherings and celebrations in strengthening family ties across generations.

9.17 Exploring Therapeutic Modalities for Emotional Well-being

Therapeutic modalities tailored to the unique needs of seniors can significantly contribute to emotional well-being. This section explores various therapeutic approaches and interventions designed to support seniors in addressing emotional challenges.

- **Art and Music Therapy:**
    - The therapeutic benefits of art and music therapy in promoting emotional expression and well-being.
    - Incorporating creative modalities into therapeutic interventions for seniors.

- **Reminiscence Therapy:**
    - Exploring reminiscence therapy as a valuable approach for seniors to reflect on positive memories and life experiences.
    - Creating opportunities for seniors to share and celebrate their personal histories.

- **Animal-Assisted Therapy:**
    - The positive effects of animal-assisted therapy on emotional well-being, including reduced stress and increased feelings of companionship.
    - Collaborating with therapy animals and trained professionals to incorporate animal-assisted interventions.

9.18 Cultivating a Positive and Supportive Living Environment

The physical environment plays a crucial role in influencing seniors' mental and emotional well-being. This section explores strategies for creating a positive and supportive living environment that enhances their overall quality of life.

- **Designing Senior-Friendly Spaces:**
    - Adapting living spaces to be senior-friendly, considering factors such as accessibility, safety, and comfort.
    - Collaborating with design professionals to enhance the functionality and aesthetics of

living environments.

- **Community Engagement and Inclusivity:**
  - Promoting community engagement and inclusivity to combat social isolation and enhance seniors' sense of belonging.
  - The importance of accessible public spaces and community initiatives that cater to seniors.

- **Respectful and Person-Centered Care:**
  - Advocating for person-centered care that respects seniors' preferences, autonomy, and individuality.
  - Training caregivers and healthcare professionals in providing empathetic and respectful care.

9.19 Coping with Grief and Loss in Later Life

Grief and loss are inevitable aspects of later life, and seniors may face challenges in coping with the loss of loved ones, health, or independence. This section explores strategies for supporting seniors through the grieving process and providing compassionate care.

- **Understanding the Grieving Process:**
  - Recognizing the stages of grief and the unique ways in which seniors may experience loss.
  - The importance of allowing individuals to grieve in their own time and manner.

- **Grief Support Services:**
  - The availability of grief support services, including counseling, support groups, and community resources.
  - Collaborating with professionals experienced in grief and bereavement to provide tailored support.

- **Creating Rituals and Commemorative Practices:**
  - Encouraging the creation of rituals and commemorative practices to honor and remember loved ones.
  - The healing potential of meaningful ceremonies and tributes in the grieving process.

9.20 Evaluating Mental and Emotional Well-being: Continuous Monitoring and Adjustments

The chapter concludes by emphasizing the importance of continuous monitoring and adjustments to support seniors' mental and emotional well-being over time.

- **Regular Assessments and Check-ins:**
  - The role of regular assessments and check-ins to monitor seniors' mental and emotional health.
  - Collaborating with healthcare providers, caregivers, and mental health professionals to identify emerging challenges.

- **Adapting Supportive Interventions:**
  - Strategies for adapting supportive interventions based on changes in seniors' needs, preferences, and life circumstances.
  - The flexibility of care plans to address evolving mental and emotional well-being requirements.

- **Holistic and Person-Centered Care:**
  - Reinforcing the importance of holistic and person-centered approaches to mental and emotional well-being.
  - Collaborating across disciplines to provide comprehensive and tailored care for seniors.

In conclusion, prioritizing mental and emotional well-being is essential for seniors to lead fulfilling lives. By implementing strategies that address cognitive vitality, emotional resilience, social connections, and the creation of supportive environments, communities, caregivers, and healthcare professionals can contribute to the holistic well-being of seniors in their later years.

CHAPTER 10: SPIRITUAL AND MEANINGFUL LIVING IN LATER LIFE

As individuals age, the pursuit of spiritual and meaningful living becomes increasingly significant. This chapter explores the diverse dimensions of spirituality, the search for meaning, and how seniors can cultivate a sense of purpose, connection, and transcendence in their later years.

10.1 Understanding the Role of Spirituality

Spirituality, often intertwined with religious beliefs but not limited to them, plays a crucial role in the lives of many seniors. This section delves into the multifaceted nature of spirituality and its impact on overall well-being.

- **Defining Spirituality in Later Life:**
  - Recognizing spirituality as a personal and evolving aspect of identity.
  - Distinguishing between organized religion and individual spiritual experiences.

- **Spirituality and Quality of Life:**
  - Exploring the correlation between spirituality and improved quality of life among seniors.
  - The role of spiritual practices in providing comfort, resilience, and a sense of purpose.

- **Inclusivity of Different Belief Systems:**
  - Acknowledging and respecting diverse spiritual beliefs, including Christianity, Islam, Buddhism, Hinduism, and various non-religious spiritual perspectives.

- Fostering an inclusive environment that allows seniors to explore and express their spiritual identity.

10.2 The Search for Meaning in Later Life

The quest for meaning is a fundamental aspect of the human experience, and in later life, individuals often engage in introspection and reflection to find deeper significance. This section explores the search for meaning and strategies for cultivating a sense of purpose.

- **Life Reflection and Legacy:**
    - Encouraging seniors to engage in life reflection and consider the legacy they want to leave.
    - The impact of contemplating one's life journey on finding meaning and purpose.

- **Identifying Personal Values:**
    - Exploring personal values and how they contribute to a meaningful life.
    - The alignment of daily actions with core values for a sense of authenticity and purpose.

- **Contributing to Others and Society:**
    - The fulfillment derived from contributing to the well-being of others and society.
    - Strategies for identifying opportunities for volunteerism, mentorship, and community engagement.

10.3 The Role of Rituals and Ceremonies

Rituals and ceremonies hold cultural, spiritual, and personal significance, providing a framework for expressing beliefs, celebrating milestones, and finding solace. This section explores the importance of rituals in later life.

- **Religious and Cultural Ceremonies:**
    - Participating in religious ceremonies and cultural rituals that hold personal significance.
    - The role of traditions in fostering a sense of continuity and connection with the past.
- **Personal Rituals for Reflection:**
    - Creating personal rituals for reflection, meditation, or prayer.
    - The meditative and grounding aspects of daily or periodic rituals.
- **Celebratory Rituals for Milestones:**
    - Developing celebratory rituals for birthdays, anniversaries, and other life milestones.
    - The joy and sense of achievement derived from acknowledging personal and shared accomplishments.

10.4 Mindfulness and Presence in the Moment

The practice of mindfulness, rooted in various spiritual traditions, has gained prominence for its positive impact on mental well-being. This section explores how seniors can embrace mindfulness to enhance their connection with the present moment.

- **Mindful Awareness Practices:**
    - Incorporating mindful awareness practices, such as meditation and deep breathing exercises, into daily routines.
    - The benefits of mindfulness in reducing stress, enhancing focus, and fostering a sense of peace.
- **Gratitude and Appreciation:**
    - Cultivating gratitude as a mindful practice to appreciate the small joys in life.

- Expressing gratitude for relationships, experiences, and the richness of the present moment.

- **Nature and Mindful Connection:**
    - Engaging in nature-based mindfulness activities, such as mindful walks or contemplation in natural settings.
    - The restorative and spiritual aspects of connecting with the natural world.

10.5 Spiritual Communities and Fellowship

Many seniors find spiritual support and companionship through involvement in religious or spiritual communities. This section explores the benefits of spiritual fellowship and the sense of belonging it provides.

- **Community Worship and Services:**
    - Participating in community worship services and religious gatherings.
    - The communal aspects of shared rituals, prayers, and spiritual teachings.

- **Supportive Networks and Friendship:**
    - Building supportive networks and friendships within spiritual communities.
    - The role of shared values and beliefs in fostering deep connections.

- **Interfaith Dialogue and Understanding:**
    - Encouraging interfaith dialogue to promote understanding and respect among individuals from diverse spiritual backgrounds.
    - The potential for shared values and common goals in fostering unity.

10.6 Holistic Wellness and the Integration of Spirituality

Spirituality is integral to holistic wellness, encompassing physical, mental, emotional, and spiritual dimensions. This section explores the integration of spirituality into comprehensive wellness practices.

- **Spirituality and Physical Health:**
    - Exploring the connections between spirituality and physical well-being.
    - The potential positive impact of spiritual practices on immune function, cardiovascular health, and overall vitality.

- **Mind-Body-Spirit Integration:**
    - Embracing holistic wellness by integrating spiritual practices with mental and emotional well-being.
    - The interconnectedness of mind, body, and spirit in fostering overall health.

- **Spiritual Guidance in Health Decisions:**
    - Considering spiritual beliefs and values in health decisions and medical treatments.
    - Collaboration between healthcare providers and spiritual leaders to ensure holistic care.

10.7 Facing End-of-life Issues with Spiritual Resilience

Navigating end-of-life issues is a profound aspect of later life, and spirituality often plays a significant role in providing comfort, guidance, and resilience. This section explores how seniors can face end-of-life issues with spiritual strength.

- **Spiritual Coping Strategies:**
    - Identifying spiritual coping strategies to navigate existential concerns and fears related to death.

- The role of faith, prayer, and spiritual support in finding solace.

- **Advance Spiritual Care Planning:**
    - Engaging in advance spiritual care planning to address spiritual preferences and rituals at the end of life.
    - Collaborating with spiritual leaders and caregivers to ensure meaningful end-of-life experiences.

- **Spiritual Support for Grieving and Loss:**
    - Seeking spiritual support and rituals for coping with grief and loss.
    - The transformative potential of spiritual practices in the healing journey.

10.8 Exploring Transcendence and Connection to the Divine

The search for transcendence and connection to the divine is a central aspect of spiritual exploration. This section delves into how seniors can nurture a sense of transcendence and connect with the divine in their later years.

- **Contemplative Practices for Transcendence:**
    - Engaging in contemplative practices, such as prayer or meditation, to experience moments of transcendence.
    - The potential for spiritual experiences to provide a sense of awe, wonder, and connection.

- **Sacred Spaces and Rituals:**
    - Creating sacred spaces for personal reflection, meditation, or prayer.
    - Incorporating sacred rituals that facilitate a sense of connection to the divine.

- **Interfaith Perspectives on Transcendence:**

- Exploring interfaith perspectives on transcendence and the universal human longing for connection to the divine.
- The commonalities and shared spiritual experiences across diverse religious traditions.

10.9 Integrating Technology for Spiritual Connection

Technology can serve as a valuable tool for seniors to connect with spiritual resources, communities, and teachings. This section explores how technology can enhance spiritual experiences in later life.

- **Virtual Spiritual Communities:**
  - Engaging in virtual spiritual communities through online services, discussions, and events.
  - The accessibility and inclusivity of virtual platforms for seniors with mobility or transportation challenges.
- **Spiritual Apps and Resources:**
  - Exploring spiritual apps and online resources that provide guided meditations, scripture readings, and inspirational content.
  - Tailoring technology usage to enhance spiritual practices and connections.
- **Virtual Pilgrimages and Retreats:**
  - Participating in virtual pilgrimages and retreats to sacred sites or spiritual destinations.
  - The potential for technology to bring transformative spiritual experiences into the homes of seniors.

10.10 Legacy Building and Spiritual Reflection

As seniors reflect on their lives, legacy building becomes

a meaningful endeavor. This section explores how spiritual reflection can contribute to the creation of a legacy that aligns with one's values and beliefs.

- **Documenting Spiritual Journeys:**
    - Documenting spiritual journeys, reflections, and insights for future generations.
    - The potential for spiritual narratives to inspire and guide others on their own paths.

- **Creating Sacred Artifacts:**
    - Crafting sacred artifacts or symbols that represent one's spiritual beliefs and legacy.
    - The tangible and symbolic value of creating items infused with personal spirituality.

- **Sharing Spiritual Wisdom:**
    - Sharing spiritual wisdom, teachings, and experiences with family, friends, and communities.
    - The intergenerational transmission of spiritual values and insights.

10.11 Cultural Sensitivity and Respect for Diverse Beliefs

In addressing spiritual needs, it is essential to approach each individual with cultural sensitivity and respect for diverse beliefs. This section emphasizes the importance of recognizing and honoring the unique spiritual perspectives of seniors from various cultural backgrounds.

- **Cultural Competence in Spiritual Care:**
    - Providing culturally competent spiritual care that respects diverse belief systems, traditions, and practices.
    - Collaborating with spiritual leaders who are familiar with the cultural nuances of diverse communities.

- **Open Dialogue on Spirituality:**
    - Encouraging open dialogue on spirituality to understand individual beliefs, values, and preferences.
    - Creating an inclusive and non-judgmental space for seniors to express their spiritual identities.
- **Respecting Non-religious Spirituality:**
    - Acknowledging and respecting non-religious or secular forms of spirituality.
    - Providing support for seniors who may find meaning and connection through philosophy, nature, or personal reflections.

10.12 Engaging in Intergenerational Spiritual Experiences

Interactions with younger generations provide opportunities for seniors to share their spiritual wisdom and learn from the perspectives of the younger demographic. This section explores intergenerational spiritual experiences and the mutual enrichment that occurs.

- **Sharing Spiritual Stories:**
    - Sharing personal spiritual stories with younger family members, fostering intergenerational understanding.
    - The potential for shared spiritual narratives to strengthen family bonds.
- **Mentorship and Spiritual Guidance:**
    - Serving as spiritual mentors or guides for younger individuals seeking wisdom and guidance.
    - The reciprocal nature of mentorship, with both seniors and younger generations benefiting from shared experiences.

- **Participating in Intergenerational Spiritual Activities:**
  - Engaging in intergenerational spiritual activities, such as attending religious services, rituals, or discussions together.
  - Building bridges between generations through shared spiritual experiences.

10.13 Spiritual Resilience in Times of Adversity

Spiritual resilience is a source of strength that can help seniors navigate challenging times and find meaning in adversity. This section explores how spiritual beliefs and practices contribute to resilience.

- **Finding Meaning in Adversity:**
  - Drawing on spiritual beliefs to find meaning and purpose in the face of adversity.
  - The transformative potential of reframing challenges through a spiritual lens.

- **Prayer and Meditation as Coping Mechanisms:**
  - Using prayer and meditation as coping mechanisms to navigate stress, grief, and loss.
  - The calming and centering effects of spiritual practices during difficult times.

- **Community Support and Spiritual Networks:**
  - Seeking support from spiritual communities and networks during times of adversity.
  - The strength derived from shared spiritual values and a sense of belonging.

10.14 Encouraging Dialogue on Spirituality in Healthcare Settings

In healthcare settings, recognizing and addressing the spiritual needs of seniors is integral to providing holistic care. This section explores the importance of open dialogue on spirituality within healthcare environments.

- **Training Healthcare Professionals:**
  - Providing training for healthcare professionals on recognizing and addressing spiritual needs.
  - The role of spiritual care teams in comprehensive healthcare settings.

- **Spiritual Assessment and Care Plans:**
  - Incorporating spiritual assessments into overall care plans to tailor support to individual beliefs.
  - Collaboration between healthcare providers and spiritual leaders to enhance patient-centered care.

- **Respecting End-of-life Spiritual Wishes:**
  - Ensuring that end-of-life spiritual wishes are respected and integrated into care plans.
  - Facilitating open communication between healthcare providers, patients, and their spiritual communities.

10.15 Future Trends in Spiritual Living for Seniors

The chapter concludes by exploring emerging trends in spiritual living for seniors. Anticipating future developments allows for proactive adaptation and enhancement of spiritual support programs.

- **Virtual Reality Spiritual Experiences:**
  - The potential integration of virtual reality for immersive spiritual experiences, such as virtual pilgrimages or meditative environments.
  - Utilizing technology to create accessible and transformative spiritual encounters.

- **Innovations in Spiritual Care Training:**

- Advancements in training programs for healthcare professionals and caregivers in providing culturally sensitive and spiritually informed care.

- The integration of diverse spiritual perspectives into educational curricula.

- **Global Perspectives on Elder Spirituality:**
    - A growing recognition of global perspectives on elder spirituality, with an emphasis on cross-cultural understanding and collaboration.

    - Exchange programs and initiatives that facilitate the sharing of spiritual wisdom across diverse communities.

- **Interfaith and Intergenerational Dialogues:**
    - The promotion of interfaith and intergenerational dialogues to foster mutual understanding, respect, and shared spiritual experiences.

    - Initiatives that bring together individuals from different faith traditions and age groups for meaningful conversations.

In conclusion, Chapter 10 emphasizes the significance of spiritual and meaningful living in later life. By exploring diverse dimensions of spirituality, understanding the search for meaning, and integrating spiritual practices into holistic wellness, seniors can navigate their later years with a sense of purpose, connection, and transcendence. The chapter highlights the importance of cultural sensitivity, intergenerational connections, and ongoing dialogue on spirituality in creating supportive environments that nurture the spiritual well-being of seniors.

CHAPTER 11: SUMMARY OF "PROMOTING SAFETY AND WELL-BEING FOR SENIORS AT HOME"

As we conclude our journey through the pages of this book, it's essential to reflect on the wealth of information and insights shared to enhance the safety and well-being of seniors at home. Throughout the chapters, we've delved into critical aspects of senior care, starting with the importance of home safety assessments and fall prevention strategies. We've underscored the necessity of adapting homes to meet seniors' evolving needs, ensuring their living environments remain conducive to their health and mobility. Addressing cognitive health emerged as a crucial focal point, with recommendations ranging from cognitive exercises to fostering social connections to maintain mental acuity. Moreover, our exploration of emotional and spiritual well-being emphasized the significance of holistic approaches to senior care, recognizing the interconnectedness of physical, mental, and spiritual dimensions.

In summary, this book serves as a comprehensive guide, offering practical advice, evidence-based strategies, and insightful perspectives to empower seniors, caregivers, and healthcare professionals in their efforts to create safe, supportive, and fulfilling living environments for older adults. By integrating the principles outlined within these pages into everyday practices, we can collectively work towards enhancing the quality of life for seniors and ensuring they thrive in their later years. As we bid farewell to this journey, let us carry forward the knowledge gained and continue our commitment to promoting the safety, well-being, and dignity of seniors in our communities.